BASIC HEALTH PUBLICATIONS USER'S GUIDE

TO THE B-COMPLEX VITAMINS

Learn About th[...]
That Combat St[...],
Boost Energy, and
Slow the Aging
Process.

BURT BERKSON, M.D., PH.D.,
AND ARTHUR J. BERKSON, M.D.

JACK CHALLEM Series Editor

T0273406

Series Editor: Jack Challem
Editor: Carol Rosenberg
Typesetter: Gary A. Rosenberg
Series Cover Designer: Mike Stromberg

Basic Health Publications User's Guides are published by Basic Health Publications, Inc.

CONTENTS

The authors wish to thank
Rebecca Berkson
for her editing expertise
and time that she spent getting
this book into shape.

INTRODUCTION

To show you just how important B vitamins are, let's begin this User's Guide with a true story about how one of the B vitamins was used to treat a very serious condition: Ronald, a lawyer from New York City, was having difficulty concentrating on his case file. To pass the time, he watched an attractive secretary from down the hall through his office window. He knew her name was Robin, but that was all he knew about her. He decided he wanted to know her better, so that evening, he introduced himself and asked her to join him for a bite to eat. She agreed. They drove to an uptown restaurant and had a delicious dinner of prime rib with grilled wild spring mushrooms.

Later that evening, on their way up to Robin's apartment, Ronald became extremely nauseated in the elevator. Once they got into her apartment, he ran straight for the bathroom and started vomiting profusely and had a terrible case of diarrhea. Shortly thereafter, Robin also became sick with similar symptoms. They decided to get themselves to the nearest emergency room.

The attending physician asked if they'd eaten anything unusual that night. When he heard about the wild spring mushrooms, he immediately called the Centers for Disease Control in Atlanta, Georgia, and they referred him to me, Dr. Burt Berkson.

I told the ER doctor to call the restaurant for the source of the mushrooms. It turned out that the mushrooms were an imported handpicked variety from Asia. It was clear to me that the hand pickers had inadvertently gathered some poisonous mushrooms along with the harmless ones. I recommended an intravenous infusion of vitamin B_6 (pyridoxine) solution for Ronald and Robin. The infusion was administered, and Ronald and Robin survived the mushroom poisoning, if not their first date.

How did a simple B-complex vitamin save their lives? In this case, the mushroom poisoning had depleted their storehouse of vitamin B_6 (pyridoxine), an essential nutrient. (You'll learn more about vitamin B_6 in Chapter 6.)

The B vitamins can't erase one's memory of a first date gone sour, but as you'll learn in this guide, they can do many other important things for you. On any normal day in our medical office, we might use B-complex vitamins to help treat patients with high cholesterol, heart disease, headaches, poor immune function, anemia, cold sores, shingles, and genital herpes. This remarkable family of vitamins works together as a team to support the health of the entire nervous system.

The B complex family of vitamins includes vitamin B_1 (thiamine), vitamin B_2 (riboflavin), vitamin B_3 (niacin and niacinamide), vitamin B_5 (pantothenic acid), vitamin B_6 (pyridoxine), vitamin B_{12} (cobalamin), folic acid (folate), biotin, choline, inositol, and para-amino benzoic acid (PABA). Each B-complex vitamin has a fundamentally different function and a very distinct chemical structure from the others. Your body needs them all in the proper amounts and in the correct balance to stay healthy. By reading this book, you'll discover the importance of these essential substances and the impact that they have on your well-being.

When people are deficient, they are almost

never deficient in just one of the B vitamins. And since the B vitamins work best as a team, it's important to take a B-complex supplement when taking additional amounts of any single B vitamin. This promotes the natural synergism of the whole family. (Nevertheless, be sure to follow your doctor's instructions.) Some people may need to supplement with one or two of the B vitamins in particular, and most people will benefit from a daily B-complex supplement. Read on to learn how the various B vitamins can help improve your health and keep you going strong.

CHAPTER 1

THE EXTRAORDINARY B VITAMINS

B vitamins—you've probably seen them listed on cereal boxes and multivitamin labels; they're sandwiched between the more popular vitamins A and C. Most people know that vitamin A is good for the eyes and that vitamin C boosts the immune system, but what about the B vitamins? What are they good for? Probably much more than you realize. Although B vitamins have had much less media hype than antioxidants, they are certainly just as important to your physical health and mental well-being. In fact, some B vitamins, such as vitamin B_5 (pantothenic acid) and vitamin B_6 (pyridoxine) even act as antioxidants, or free-radical scavengers, and protect your cell membranes and DNA from damage.

What Are B Vitamins?

The B vitamins are a group of nutrients that are essential to the proper functioning of your blood and entire immune system. They are necessary for the transformation of food into usable energy, proper nervous system function, and good heart health, to name just a few of their important roles.

There are several distinct nutrients that are recognized as B-complex vitamins. They

Antioxidants
Compounds that obstruct, restrain, or neutralize free radicals—unstable molecules with extra electron(s) that can destroy biological substances in the body, which can lead to disease.

are all water soluble and are necessary for your body to function properly. Sometimes they work individually, but they usually work together as a team. Also, they often need to work in tandem with other molecules and different types of vitamins to function most efficiently.

Even though they are water soluble, some B vitamins can be stored in the body. Others are constantly consumed by chemical reactions or simply excreted through urination and, as a result, must be consumed on a daily basis. If you eat a lot of processed food, drink a lot of alcohol, take certain medications, are on a strict weight-loss diet, or are inclined to fast, you may not have sufficient amounts of one or more of the B vitamins in your body.

Vitamins
Organic substances that are found in most natural foods, or sometimes synthesized in small amounts in the body, necessary for growth and metabolism.

Although vitamins, by definition, are nutrients that cannot be manufactured by the body, some of the B vitamins are actually produced in tiny amounts in the digestive tract or in certain organs. However, this production is usually not adequate to meet the body's requirements.

Foods Rich in B Vitamins

B vitamins are found in many types of foods. They are often naturally grouped together in various combinations to help one another do their jobs. Organ meats such as liver and kidney are excellent sources of B-complex vitamins. Muscle meats, like steaks and ribs, have high levels of vitamin B_{12}, but are not otherwise a good source of B vitamins. Leafy green vegetables, whole grains, and legumes (such as beans and peas), on the other hand, are all great sources of the B-complex vitamins.

Over the past century or so, food manufacturers have been producing cereal products and breads that are highly palatable and clean looking. Disappointingly, these foods have been stripped of their bran and germ. As a result, they are also almost devoid of B-complex vitamins. Due to this process, naturally occurring B-complex vitamins are almost absent from most white breads, pastas, breakfast cereals, and other foods made of simple, highly processed carbohydrates. While most manufacturers add exogenous B vitamins (B vitamins from other sources) to their products, these are not in the perfect balance that nature intended.

Are You Getting Enough B Vitamins?

Most adults could probably benefit from taking up to three times or more the recommended daily allowances (RDAs) of many of the B vitamins. The RDA values were calculated more than sixty years ago during World War II. Their original purpose was not to maximize health and nutrition, but to provide the minimum amounts necessary to avoid flagrant diseases of vitamin deficiency such as pellagra (niacin deficiency) and beriberi (thiamine deficiency).

Recommended Daily Allowances (RDAs)

The minimum amounts of vitamins and minerals necessary to avoid serious deficiencies.

Vitamin B Deficiency

The signs and symptoms of early vitamin deficiency are often more elusive and subtle than those of the major diseases. They can include fatigue, tingling in your fingers and toes (paresthesia), paleness, and even a painful inflamed tongue (glossitis), among other signs. Experiencing any one of these symptoms may signal that you are heading for a serious B-vitamin deficiency. While malnourished people in underdeveloped countries may exhibit obvious signs and symptoms of flagrant B-vitamin deficiency, even people in highly developed societies such as the United States are susceptible to vitamin deficiencies.

The reason for this is multifactorial. For one thing, just the act of cooking food can destroy the structure and function of several of the B vitamins and, therefore, their potency. That's why it's best to include some well-washed fresh raw foods in your diet, including leafy green vegetables, broccoli, cauliflower, cabbage, and green beans.

Also, many of us simply eat a diet that is lacking the B vitamins we need. In general, we depend on simple carbohydrates (sugars and starches), refined bakery goods, and fast foods for a large part of our daily calorie intake. As mentioned earlier, these foods are stripped of their natural vitamins during processing. Then, the nutrients are often added back in suboptimal combinations, quality, and quantity, to arrive at a final product that is not conducive to good health. It is much healthier to eat natural foods, such as whole grains and beans, than to eat highly processed foods, such as packaged muffins and canned refried beans. Here's a good rule of thumb: the more a food resembles it original state from the earth, the healthier it is.

Another reason some of us may become deficient has to do with the use of antibiotics. The beneficial bacteria that reside in the large intestines are responsible for producing small amounts of B vitamins in the body. However, when you take a course of certain antibiotics, the antibiotics kill not only the "dangerous" bacteria that may be causing disease but the beneficial bacteria as well. So, as a result, you may become relatively vitamin deficient. Therefore, it's important to replace your intestinal bacteria by taking a high-quality probiotic (good bacteria) supplement, such as acidophilus, or by eating unprocessed yogurt with live cultures for the entire course of the antibiotic regimen and for the following two weeks.

For all these reasons, chances are you can benefit from supplementing your diet with a high-quality B-complex capsule. (We recommend capsules over tablets, since tablets are produced under heat and pressure, which destroy some B vitamins.)

B Vitamins Offer Protection

While being deficient in B vitamins can lead to a state of disharmony and disease, carefully supplementing your diet with B vitamins can help protect you from other diseases. Researchers have shown that B vitamins have roles ranging from protection against heart disease and various forms of cancer to improvement in mood disorders. They perform these functions in many different ways. Let's take a closer look.

B Vitamins and Heart Health

One way in which B vitamins protect you from heart disease is tied to the amino acid homocysteine, which is produced by the body during the breakdown of protein. Research has repeatedly shown that an increased level of homocysteine in the blood is an important risk factor for serious damage to arteries, which can lead to heart disease and strokes.

Several studies illustrate the beneficial effects of B vitamins on homocysteine levels. For example, in one study, homocysteine levels were significantly lowered in more than 600 patients with B-vitamin supplementation. The three key B vitamins that were shown to effectively reduce homocysteine levels are folic acid, vitamin B_6, and vitamin B_{12}. The lowering of homocysteine levels and the reduction of cardiovascular risk was shown to occur at doses of approximately 400 micrograms (mcg) of folic acid, 7 milligrams (mg) of vitamin B_6 per day, and 400 mcg of vitamin B_{12}.

B Vitamins and Cancer Prevention

The antioxidant properties of certain B vitamins can potentially offer your body protection against cancer. Most cancers begin with a mutation, or random change, in deoxyribonucleic acid (DNA)—the body's genetic blueprint. A lack of folic acid interferes with DNA's ability to repair its own damage. It is the accumulation of such damage that underlies the causes of aging and cancer. In a recent Australian study, scientists found that supplementing a diet with high amounts of folic acid and vitamin B_{12} lowered levels of chromosomal damage in otherwise healthy young adults.

"B" Well and Happy

The B vitamins also have a long history as anti-stress nutrients and mood enhancers. This is not surprising because B-complex vitamins are essential for healthy brain function. Several scientists theorize that the initial signs of B-vitamin deficiency are irritability and difficulty dealing with stress. Along these lines, psychological studies have shown that providing college students with high-potency vitamins improves their mood and demeanor.

What's the Right Dose for You?

It is not possible to give you a specific prescription for your daily doses of B-complex vitamins. This is because every person—depending on age, body weight, diet, exercise habits, health status, occupation, sex, and levels of mental and physical stress—requires a tailored B-complex vitamin regimen. A reputable and knowledgeable integrative or naturopathic doctor can design such a program for you. Health food stores and pharmacies generally carry an assortment of B-complex vitamins in various dosages; ask for assistance in selecting the appropriate one for you.

For our own purposes, we've found that high-quality B-complex capsules in the formulation listed below, taken twice daily, suits our needs:

- 25 mg of thiamine (vitamin B_1)

- 25 mg of riboflavin (vitamin B_2)

- 150 mg of niacin (vitamin B_3) as mixed niacinamide and niacin

- 150 mg of pantothenic acid (vitamin B_5)

- 55 mg of pyridoxine (vitamin B_6)

- 400 mcg of vitamin B_{12}

- 800 mcg of folic acid

- 400 mcg biotin

- 50 mg choline

- 50 mg inositol

- 50 mg PABA

If a virus is brewing, we may double this dose. (There's more on viral infections in Chapter 5.) In addition to this B-complex supplement, we take 300 mg of alpha-lipoic acid (of European origin) and 200 mg of coenzyme Q_{10}. Both alpha-lipoic acid (see Chapter 11) and coenzyme Q_{10} are good antioxidants and assist the body in producing energy. Another important antioxidant, which we include in our supplement regimen, is vitamin E (400 IU of mixed tocopherols). This vitamin neutralizes free radicals in cell membranes and fatty tissues. We also take 25,000 IU of beta-carotene and 200 mcg of natural selenium. We often recommend these additional supplements to our patients as well.

In addition to this regimen, we maintain a healthy diet that includes at least six servings of green vegetables each day, as well as an exercise regimen that includes weight training and jogging. Since we have been on this health program, we feel great. With a healthy diet and exercise, and a vitamin regimen that includes B vitamins, you will surely feel great too.

Keep This in Mind

Despite all the benefits of the B vitamins, keep in mind that any substance can be toxic in extremely high doses, even water. So, be sure not to overdose on B vitamins. Also, since these vitamins have so many interrelated functions, they should be taken together in a high-quality B-complex capsule. Taking too much of one individual B vitamin for too long can suppress the activity of other B vitamins, thereby causing a disruption in the body. This disruption can lead to disease. If, after reading this book, you believe you need higher doses of a single B vitamin, be sure to consult a knowledgeable healthcare practitioner. Also, be sure to take a B-complex supplement for additional dietary support.

CHAPTER 2

VITAMIN B$_1$
(THIAMINE)

Vitamin B$_1$ (thiamine), a water-soluble compound like all the other B vitamins, is a coenzyme that helps the body's biochemical catalysts, or enzymes, do their jobs to speed up the chemical reactions that power our biological functions. When you eat, the food's energy is converted to an important substance called "pyruvate." Pyruvate is full of energy but cannot enter the mitochondria (the energy-producing factories of the cells) for processing. It must first be converted to acetyl coenzyme A, which is the fuel for your mitochondria. This conversion requires an ample supply of vitamin B$_1$ and other substances such as alpha-lipoic acid (see Chapter 11).

Enzyme
A protein produced by the body that acts as a catalyst in biochemical reactions.

Thiamine is also necessary for digestion and blood-cell formation, and aids in the breakdown of alcohol into harmless end products, specifically carbon dioxide and water, which the body can easily excrete. Additionally, thiamine appears to help hold connective tissues together. Known for its antistress properties, it's also critical for proper function of the adrenal glands, which produce hormones that regulate mental, physical, and immunological stress in the body. Studies have shown that, without enough thiamine, animals can develop adrenal tumors or suppressed immune-system function, making them more susceptible to infections.

Thiamine is also important to the nervous system. It is required for the production of acetylcholine, a neurotransmitter, which passes important messages from one nerve cell to the next. In the cardiovascular system, thiamine—acting together with other substances—may reduce the formation of arterial plaques that can lead to heart attacks and strokes.

Neurotransmitter *Chemicals that pass messages from one nerve cell to another.*

Lastly, thiamine has been shown to have therapeutic effects in people with chronic fatigue, Alzheimer's disease, Bell's palsy, and diabetes. In fact, we've only scratched the surface of the many functions thiamine has in the body.

Sources of Thiamine

This vitamin is found in relatively high amounts in whole grains (when all the parts of the grain are intact). Whole cereal grains, such as oatmeal and buckwheat, are good sources of thiamine. Other foods that contain high levels of thiamine are brown rice, egg yolks, fresh beans, fish, brewer's yeast, and pork. Vitamin B_1 is easily destroyed by heat, so overcooking should be avoided. (Keep in mind, however, not to *undercook* pork, fish, or egg yolks.)

Thiamine Deficiency

What are the consequences of not eating sufficient amounts of vitamin B_1? Here is an extreme example: During World War II, prisoners of war in Asia were fed a diet consisting almost entirely of white rice. As a result, many of them became very ill with symptoms that included diarrhea, swollen abdomens, fatigue, and weight loss. In severe instances, some prisoners experienced heart failure and severe nerve damage that, in some cases, led to paralysis. This constellation of symptoms defines the disease known as "beriberi." A 1997 study examined other disease conditions found in prisoners of concentration camps that may have been associated with thiamine deficiency, including salivary gland cysts, inguinal hernias (protrusions of part of the intestine through the groin muscles), and carpal tunnel syndrome.

Beriberi
A disease caused by a severe deficiency in thiamine that affects many systems of the body, including the muscles, heart, nerves, and digestive system.

So, why did these prisoners develop beriberi? During the processing of natural brown rice to shiny carbohydrate-rich white rice, most of the bran and germ is stripped away, and with it, all the vitamin B_1 is destroyed. As a result, the previously healthy grains of rice become an empty-calorie food entirely devoid of vitamin B_1. While this is an extreme example, we can learn a lot from what happened to the prisoners. Through our modern process of food production, many of the foods we eat are stripped of their important nutrients. That's why it's so important to eat foods as close to their original form as possible.

How can you recognize if you are thiamine deficient? Your first symptoms would most likely be fatigue, poor memory, abdominal pains, and constipation. Later, you might experience heart palpitations, paresthesias ("pins and needles") in your feet and hands, muscle weakness, and vision problems. These symptoms may indicate a serious health problem that should be checked out by a doctor. If they are found to be the result of a vitamin deficiency, supplementation should be prescribed.

While it's true that a severe deficiency of thiamine is pretty rare in developed countries such as the United States, the stresses we often expose ourselves to (smoking, drinking excessive amounts of alcohol, and eating lots of junk foods) can deplete the amount of, and increase the need for, thiamine. Smoking, for instance, causes a buildup of toxic products, or free radicals, that tear apart your tissues and DNA. Since vitamin B_1 also functions as an antioxidant, it can help protect you from the destructive effects of free radicals.

Alcoholism and Thiamine

Because the body requires thiamine to break down alcohol, alcoholism directly causes a lack of thiamine in the body. The more alcohol a person drinks, the more thiamine his or her body uses up. Moreover, people who drink excessive amounts of alcohol on a regular basis typically have a poor diet. This compounds their thiamine-deficient state. If excessive drinking continues, they could develop beriberi-type heart disease, permanent neurological damage, and quite possibly even die.

How Much Thiamine Is Enough?

Small amounts of vitamin B_1 are stored in the liver and kidneys, but you should still aim to get some thiamine from your diet on a daily basis. (Any excess is eliminated in your urine and perspiration.) In general, thiamine should be taken as part of a B-complex vitamin capsule. In an ideal world, each person would take a tailored amount of thiamine to meet his or her needs, and that amount would certainly exceed the government's recommendations. The RDA for adults is very low at 1.5 mg per day. We personally take 50–100 mg of thiamine a day, which seems to be a suitable amount. This is obviously a significant difference. We feel it's the difference between barely preventing beriberi and maximizing our health. Many nutritionally oriented doctors often use thiamine with a balance of other supplements, including a B-complex vitamin, to treat chronic fatigue as well as depression and lack of self-esteem, with this dosage range.

Many of our patients who have increased their thiamine intake—along with a balance of other vitamins and increased physical activity—feel an enormous increase in energy. Also, if you're an active person, you may require much more thiamine than a sedentary person, since body stores of thiamine are not very large and can be used up quickly with the elevated metabolism of an active person.

Thiamine Intake in the Elderly

Thiamine intake is especially important in the elderly. As we get older, our bodies generally have less of this vitamin. In one study, doctors in Belgium reported that geriatric patients have only about 50 percent of the amount of thiamine in their brains that infants have. Similarly, about half of all nursing home patients have been found to have low thiamine levels. Also, a group of researchers in Toronto reported that thiamine supplementation provided modest improvement in the brain function of people with Alzheimer's disease, an age-related disease.

Thiamine's Effects on Mood and Mental Function

Many of our patients have reported that thiamine supplementation improves their mood and sharpens their mental functioning. Other doctors have received similar reports. For example, Dr. David Benton of the University of Wales gave thiamine to a group of volunteers with depression. He found that they became more clear-headed, energetic, and self-composed after three months of treatment. Another research group from the United Kingdom studied the long-term effect of vitamin supplementation on more than

120 adults. They found that enhanced thiamine status improved performance on a wide variety of cognitive function tests in women. (This improvement was not seen in the men in the study.)

Thiamine's Effects on Bell's Palsy

Bell's palsy is a relatively common condition in which one side of the face droops. When this happens, people often fear the worst—that they've had a stroke, for instance. If these symptoms do occur, a person should see his or her doctor immediately for a diagnosis. Bell's palsy is caused by partial paralysis of the facial nerve from an injury to the nerve. This injury is often precipitated by emotional stress and may be caused by a viral infection of this nerve. In our practice, we regularly use a variety of B vitamins for this condition—especially thiamine and pantothenic acid (vitamin B_5). Anecdotally speaking, we have found that by using these vitamins, the symptoms of Bell's palsy resolve much more quickly.

Thiamine's Effects on Diabetic Neuropathy

Diabetic neuropathy is a type of nerve damage often seen in people with longstanding diabetes. The condition starts out as a hypersensitivity to light touch. In advanced stages, it causes burning or electric-like piercing pains in the extremities, especially in the feet. This pain is often disabling.

A lot of doctors try to suppress the pain with medications that often don't work or lead to unsatisfactory pain relief. More enlightened doctors treat the source of this pain, the diabetes, along with relieving the symptoms. They put their patients on strict but sensible diets as well as a reasonable exercise program and usually need to use prescription medications to reach diabetic goals. Some doctors additionally prescribe vitamins and antioxidants to further aid in the diabetic care.

The use of thiamine, along with alpha-lipoic acid, encourages the blood vessels and nerves of the skin to use sugar more efficiently. With this type of natural treatment, many patients become free of pain after only a short time.

Conclusion

It should be clear now just how important thiamine is to good health. A deficiency in this vitamin can cause a spectrum of health conditions, from the subtle symptom of fatigue to the striking disease of beriberi. You can maximize your thiamine intake by eating thiamine-rich foods such as whole grains, fish, and legumes, and by taking a B-complex capsule daily.

CHAPTER 3

VITAMIN B$_2$
(RIBOFLAVIN)

Vitamin B$_2$ (riboflavin) is a distinctively fluorescent yellow molecule attached to an alcohol molecule called "ribital." (The root word "flavin" means "yellow.") Like vitamin B$_1$, riboflavin is essential for sustaining life. It is a fundamental component of a molecule called flavin adenine dinucleotide (FAD), which the body needs to produce energy.

Flavin Adenine Dinucleotide (FAD)

An enzyme required for energy production that contains one or more metals such as molybdenum or iron and is sometimes referred to as a metalo-flavoprotein.

Like thiamine, riboflavin is necessary for the operation of certain chemical cycles that produce energy. As you know, the body converts food to energy. To a large part, this energy is stored in the form of a molecule called ATP. This molecule acts like the gasoline to power your body. Riboflavin is needed for the construction of at least two fundamental coenzymes required for ATP synthesis. Without riboflavin, your cells could not effectively use oxygen or store energy. Thus, this vitamin is required for the life of your cells.

Sources of Riboflavin

Organ meats, such as liver, kidney, and pancreas, are some of the best sources of riboflavin. Perhaps even better sources are certain types of algae and brewer's yeast. Some cereals, breads, and other foods have been fortified with very small doses of riboflavin, but natural sources are, of course, best.

Riboflavin is more heat resistant than thiamine, so it does not break down as easily during cooking. It is, however, very sensitive to light. Therefore, foods and supplements containing vitamin B_2 should be stored in dark places like the refrigerator or in a cabinet. Most dairy companies have replaced glass milk bottles with waxed opaque containers to protect the riboflavin content of the milk.

Riboflavin Deficiency

To show you just how vital riboflavin is to maintaining health, we'll describe the condition ariboflavinosis, which occurs when there is a vitamin B_2 deficiency. People with this condition often complain of weakness, sore throat, crusty material at the corners of their mouths (chelosis), painful mouths, sore red tongues, and eye problems. (Chelosis is characteristic of riboflavin deficiency, but it can also be caused by a shortage of other B vitamins.) At times people with ariboflavinosis may suffer from a serious type of anemia due to poor red-blood-cell production in the bone marrow.

What can cause this kind of severe deficiency? In the underdeveloped world, scant and severely vitamin-deficient diets can lead to a severe riboflavin deficiency. But even developed countries are not immune to deficiency. People with anorexia and teenagers who follow extremely low-fat diets are at risk for low levels of vitamin B_2. Smokers are at risk for low levels of riboflavin as well: A recent medical journal article reported that male smokers had lower levels of riboflavin than their nonsmoking counterparts, suggesting that cigarette smoking may actually deplete this vitamin.

In general, a poor diet and deficiencies of

other nutrients may signal a possible deficiency of vitamin B_2.

How Much Riboflavin Is Enough?

The RDA for riboflavin is 1.7 mg. We believe this is a rather low dosage. A general recommended daily dosage of riboflavin is 10–25 mg, as part of a complete B-complex supplement. Higher doses will most likely be needed to treat riboflavin deficiency or disease, but they should only be taken under the guidance of a health-care professional.

Often, when people take riboflavin or B-complex supplements, they notice that their urine develops a fluorescent-yellow glow. This suggests that your body has used the amount of riboflavin that it needs and is excreting the rest. It does not mean that the riboflavin is not being absorbed.

Riboflavin's Effects on Migraines

Riboflavin has many possible therapeutic benefits. One extremely common condition that riboflavin may help is migraine headaches. Studies have shown that about half of the migraine sufferers who were given a short course of riboflavin (400 mg per day) experienced improvement in their condition. In one double-blind research study, high doses of riboflavin significantly decreased the frequency of headaches in eighty migraine patients over a period of one year. Although riboflavin won't reverse migraines, it is very likely a good preventative measure to take, and it lacks the side effects associated with commonly used migraine medications.

The reason that riboflavin may be effective in preventing migraines is probably tied into the role of mitochondria, the energy-producing microfactories of the body. Some scientists believe that mitochondria that are not operating efficiently can lead to migraine headaches. Riboflavin can help ramp up the energy production of mitochondria and consequently can help prevent migraine headaches.

Riboflavin's Effects on Cancer Treatment

It's a well-known fact that free-radical injury can cause severe damage to the cells and that this damage can incite the changes that cause cancer. It's also well known that antioxidants can mop up or neutralize the damage caused by the free radicals and thus prevent or control cancer. These antioxidants include vitamin C, vitamin E, alpha-lipoic acid, and coenzyme Q_{10} (CoQ_{10})—and, of course, riboflavin. Therefore, another potential therapeutic use for riboflavin is cancer prevention. For example, in a recent study, animals with laboratory-induced gene mutations that were given high dosages of riboflavin were able to repair these mutations.

In another study, a team of East Indian doctors tried to determine if combining antioxidant vitamins and prescription drugs was a more effective cancer treatment than the prescription drugs alone. Female albino rats with breast cancer were given tamoxifen, a drug often used in the chemotherapy and chemoprevention of breast cancer, along with riboflavin, niacin (vitamin B_3), and CoQ_{10} for about a month. With the administration of the combination therapy (tamoxifen plus riboflavin), the free-radical cancerous damage was restored to near normal levels. Moreover, direct antitumor activity was seen due to an increased level of a tumor-suppressor gene that makes cancer cells "go to sleep." These findings suggest that a treatment program combining standard drug therapy with antioxidant vitamins may have considerable anticancer activity and may be more effective than the ordinary drug therapy itself.

Riboflavin's Effects on Rheumatoid Arthritis

People with rheumatoid arthritis often feel worse when they are under oxidative stress (an on-slaught of free radicals). Their joints ache and swell, and over the years, can become deformed. Thus, it is important to ingest the proper amount of antioxidants to ease this problem. Additionally, scientists have reported that riboflavin supplements, which also have antioxidant activity, may help people with rheumatoid arthritis feel better. It appears that riboflavin actually helps neutralize the caustic free radicals that result in pain. In doing so, it allows for some actual healing of the injured tissues.

Oxidative Stress
Physiological stress on the body caused by free-radical damage.

Conclusion

Clearly, riboflavin is another vitally important B vitamin. While a deficiency in this vitamin results in ariboflavinosis with its varied symptoms, therapeutic doses of riboflavin have been proving to be beneficial in the treatment of migraine headaches and possibly rheumatoid arthritis. We may eventually find that this molecule has an important role in the prevention of cancer, as well. Only time and additional research will tell just how much riboflavin affects and protects our health.

CHAPTER 4

VITAMIN B₃ (NIACIN AND NIACINAMIDE)

Body tissues contain at least two forms of vitamin B₃—niacin and niacinamide. Like other B vitamins, this vitamin is also required by the body for energy production. However, it also has many exciting medical uses that range from the treatment of schizophrenia to high cholesterol. Although pure niacin and niacinamide differ slightly, the absorption and actions of both forms of this vitamin are basically the same.

Sources of Vitamin B₃

Vitamin B₃ is found in the greatest quantities in organ meats such as beef liver. Certain whole grains and legumes, such as peanuts and beans, are also good sources of this vitamin.

Niacin Deficiency

Like other B vitamins, a deficiency of niacin can lead to a disease state. The early symptoms of a niacin deficiency include weakness, a sore mouth and tongue, weight loss, and nervous irritability. If this deficiency continues, additional symptoms start to develop, including dermatitis (skin inflammation), diarrhea, and dementia (or mental confusion). These symptoms along with the proper medical tests define the diagnosis of pellagra.

Pellagra
A disease associated with niacin deficiency characterized by skin rashes, mouth sores, diarrhea, and if untreated, mental deterioration. Also known as Alpine scurvy, mal de la rosa, and Saint Ignatius' itch.

Since an inflamed digestive tract has difficulty digesting and absorbing niacin, some people will develop pellagra following a serious gastrointestinal illness or after drinking large amounts of alcohol for long periods. Also, pellagra is relatively common in many parts of the world where people consume large amounts of corn and cornmeal products. Although corn does contain niacin, its supply is tightly bound to other molecules and is, therefore, poorly digested by the intestinal tract. To make matters worse, corn contains very little tryptophan, an amino acid that the body uses to produce some niacin of its own. For this reason, pellagra was once common in the United States among poor Southerners whose diets were largely centered on cornbread. This disease actually became an epidemic in the early 1900s when crops failed and the economy started to deteriorate.

Interestingly, although Mexicans who follow a traditional diet consume a lot of cornmeal as tortillas, they do not have elevated rates of pellagra. This is because the cornmeal is first treated with limestone or wood ashes, which break the bond that keeps niacin from being digested. Beans, which contain tryptophan, are also a staple of the traditional Mexican diet, another reason why this diet does not leave one prone to niacin deficiency.

Niacin Deficiency and Cancer

Low levels of niacin for many years may predispose a person to cancer. To study this theory, a group of scientists fed animals a vitamin B_3-deficient diet. All of the animals in the study developed cancer. There are many possible reasons for this outcome. Factors involved may include niacin's relationship with the energy-carrying molecule in cells known as "nicotinamide adenine dinucleotide," or NAD, low levels of which are often see in people with cancer; niacin's role in the synthesis of coenzyme Q_{10}, which may have therapeutic effects in cancer patients; and vitamin B_3's involvement in gene repair, an essential component in the body's cancer-fighting mechanism. A better understanding of niacin metabolism will eventually lead to another piece in the cancer-prevention puzzle. It is entirely possible that niacin, in the proper amount, can be used as a cancer preventative.

How Much Vitamin B₃ Is Enough?

Vitamin B_3 is available as a supplement in two forms—niacin (or nicotinic acid) and niacinamide (or nicotinamide). The RDA for this vitamin is 15–20 mg per day. We recommend at least 50 mg of niacin and 250 mg of niacinamide daily as a maintenance dose to our average healthy adult patient. We recommend a combination of the two forms of vitamin B_3 to try and reflect how they naturally occur.

Taking a high dose of niacin for one's body size and other factors (but not niacinamide) sometimes causes a phenomenon called the "niacin flush." During this flush, there is body-wide tingling and flushing due to the release of histamine (a chemical that's released in allergic reactions and opens up blood vessels). This feeling can be frightening if it's unexpected, but it is not dangerous. Richard Kunin, M.D., of San Francisco, has shown that taking an aspirin thirty minutes prior to the niacin supplement can diminish this common side effect. Also, the flush seems to diminish with regular use of the supplement.

Niacin Flush
A harmless burning, tingling sensation in the face and chest with reddened or "flushed" skin.

Take care not to overdose on niacin. At very high doses, niacin can cause some liver damage (rarely), elevate blood sugar levels, and aggravate gout.

Niacin's Effects on Cholesterol

Abram Hoffer, M.D., Ph.D., discovered the cholesterol-lowering effect of niacin in the 1950s. Since then, it has been widely recognized among allopathic and alternative medical doctors as being an effective treatment for high cholesterol. It

---

"The Niacin Rules" for Therapeutic Use

As more information became available regarding the therapeutic use of niacin, some doctors modified Dr. Hoffer's original recommendations to make the therapy more effective. For instance, Andrew Weil, M.D., from the University of Arizona, has six "rules" for taking a therapeutic niacin regimen. They are:

1. Only use the inositol hexanicotinate form.

2. Do not use the time-release products because they are more likely to cause adverse reactions.

3. A dose of 1,000 mg should not be exceeded at any one time, and the dosing frequency should not exceed one dose every eight hours.

4. Liver function tests should be checked prior to initiating niacin therapy. They should be rechecked at regular intervals while on the program. If the liver enzymes become elevated, this suggests damage to the liver, and the niacin supplementation should be stopped immediately. The liver function will then usually return to normal in a short time.

5. Niacin should be stopped if gastrointestinal symptoms develop.

6. Cholesterol levels should be monitored monthly.

---

is even approved by the U.S. Food and Drug Administration for this purpose. In fact, many studies have shown that niacin works just as well as prescription medications at normalizing cholesterol levels without dangerous side effects.

Supplementing with niacin in doses of 200–500 mg three times a day has been shown to lower levels of "bad" cholesterol (low-density lipoproteins, or LDLs) while raising levels of "good" cholesterol (high-density lipoproteins, or HDLs). The main side effect of niacin at this level is the niacin flush. As mentioned before, the flush seems to diminish with regular use of the supplement. Julian Whitaker, M.D., a well-known medical doctor, also recommends a form of niacin called "inositol hexanicotinate" because it does not seem to cause skin flushing. (By the way, the niacinamide form of vitamin B3 also does not cause skin flushing, but it doesn't seem to have the same beneficial effect on cholesterol levels.)

Another benefit of niacin with regard to cholesterol is that it lowers the levels of lipoprotein(a) by decreasing its production in the liver. Lipoproteins are a type of cholesterol that taxis fats through the bloodstream and lymphatic system. There are various types of lipoproteins; they differ in size, composition, and density. A high level of lipoprotein(a) in particular is an important risk factor for coronary heart disease.

Niacin's Effects on Raynaud's Syndrome

Antibodies
Proteins produced by the immune system that bind to the surfaces of invading substances and microorganisms.

Raynaud's syndrome is a condition characterized by episodes of tingling, aching fingers and toes when exposed to the cold or other triggers, such as vibrations. It's caused by blood-vessel constriction and the accumulation of antibodies in the digits. This condition is sometimes seen in people with autoimmune diseases, such as scleroderma and lupus. Niacin can help this condition by acting as a vasodilator in the extremities—that is, by opening up the blood vessels and increasing blood flow to the fingers and toes.

Niacin's Effects on Mental and Neurological Disease

Both niacin and niacinamide have been used by some psychiatrists to treat serious mental and neurological conditions such as schizophrenia, epilepsy, and Parkinson's disease. Dr. Abram Hoffer pioneered the use of both niacin and niacinamide in the treatment of schizophrenia. To treat this condition, he starts most patients on 3,000 mg of niacin or niacinamide, as well as 3,000 mg of vitamin C. Because 3,000 mg is a pretty high dose, patients should have their liver enzymes regularly checked by their physicians.

Scientists have also found that vitamin B_3 supplementation decreases aggressive behavior in male animals, suggesting that it could also have the same effect in people. The hypothesis is that niacin increases the levels of the neurotransmitter serotonin, creating a feeling of calmness and well-being. Many antidepressant drugs as well as the antidepressant herb St. John's wort work by the same principle.

Conclusion

Proper niacin supplementation is not only important in preventing disease due to deficiency, but it has been shown to produce various therapeutic benefits. These benefits range from lowering "bad" cholesterol to assisting with neurological diseases. Remember, however, that there are certain caveats to taking niacin, and you should follow the "niacin rules" and talk to your doctor for safe supplementation.

CHAPTER 5

VITAMIN B$_5$
(PANTOTHENIC ACID)

Vitamin B$_5$ (pantothenic acid) is a component of one of the most important substances in your body—acetyl coenzyme A. Before the body can use sugar as fuel, it must be converted to acetyl coenzyme A. So, without pantothenic acid, your body could not produce the energy required to keep you living.

Through its interactions with other vitamins, pantothenic acid influences the way the other vitamins do their jobs. Thus, it has a wide range of functions in the body. It is involved in the production of antibodies that fight microbes and cancer. It is also part of the chain of reactions that manufacture neurotransmitters to help the brain communicate with the rest of the body. Vitamin B$_5$ also has antiviral properties, which is especially helpful during times of infection.

Sources of Pantothenic Acid

The Greek prefix "pan" means "everywhere," and true to its name, pantothenic acid is found in many natural foods. Good sources of pantothenic acid include all varieties of meats (beef, pork, chicken, and fish), whole grains, brewer's yeast, legumes (peas, beans, peanuts, and soybeans), eggs, and cabbage-type vegetables (broccoli, cauliflower, and Brussels sprouts).

Pantothenic Acid Deficiency

Pantothenic acid is easily absorbed in the intestines, so it is difficult to develop a deficiency of this B-complex vitamin. However, as we have illustrated with the other B vitamins, extra B vitamins can promote health and insufficient amounts can cause dysfunction. Similarly, if you lack sufficient amounts of pantothenic acid, you can develop symptoms of fatigue, nausea, headaches, and paresthesias ("pins and needles") in the hands and feet. A condition called "burning foot syndrome" has been identified in starving prisoners; this is thought to be related to a pantothenic-acid deficiency.

Also, as sufficient amounts of pantothenic acid can help treat and prevent viruses, insufficient amounts of pantothenic acid can leave us susceptible to outbreaks. This is illustrated in nursing homes where residents have been found to eat a diet with lower amounts of pantothenic acid and other essential nutrients than the general population. These residents are also older and often under both emotional and physical stress. As a result, they are more susceptible to all viral infections.

How Much Pantothenic Acid Is Enough?

The RDA for pantothenic acid is 4–10 mg daily. Personally, we take 500 mg daily. This amount is sufficient for most healthy people. We usually up our dosage of pantothenic acid if we feel a viral

---

Contraindication

The only contraindication to pantothenic acid supplementation is in the case of malaria. The malaria parasite (*Plasmodium*) actually requires high amounts of pantothenic acid to complete its lifecycle. In this case, high amounts of pantothenic acid in the body provide a fertile environment for the protozoan.

---

infection coming on. Extra amounts of this vitamin are also sometimes helpful or necessary during times of emotional stress.

Since pantothenic acid has many complicated interactions with a multitude of vitamins, especially those in the B-complex group, anytime you take therapeutic amounts of pantothenic acid (or any other B vitamin for that matter), it's important to also take a B-complex supplement for proper balance.

Pantothenic Acid's Effects on Wound Healing

We often prescribe this vitamin, along with zinc, vitamin C, and vitamin E for various skin lesions. These supplements, together with good wound care, usually result in decreased healing time. This may be especially important in elderly, immobile, and sick individuals (such as nursing-home residents) who are prone to vitamin deficiencies and slow-healing ulcerations on their bodies.

Pantothenic Acid's Effects on Viral Infections

Pantothenic acid is often called the "antistress vitamin" because of the role it plays in the production of stress hormones by the adrenal gland. Its role as an antistress vitamin is intricately related to why it is useful in viral infections. Most people in the world are infected by herpes-type viruses (for example, Epstein-Barr virus, shingles/chicken pox virus, and oral and genital herpes), but at any given time, the majority of those infected are not symptomatic because the viruses are usually dormant. Severe emotional or physical stress releases large amounts of stress hormones for long periods, which can cause immune-system suppression. If this occurs, any dormant virus can become active again and

Immune System
The organs, cells, and proteins that work together to protect the body from foreign substances. It includes the liver, spleen, thymus, bone marrow, and lymph system.

cause reinfection. For example, if you had chicken pox as a child, this virus normally remains dormant for the rest of your life. However, in times of high stress, the virus may become active once again, and you may develop shingles as an adult.

In our experience, outbreaks of these viral infections usually improve much faster when a person is taking higher doses of pantothenic acid. People with frequent outbreaks can use a daily dose of 500 mg per day to help prevent flare-ups. Even those with longstanding drug-resistant shingles can benefit from pantothenic acid therapy by taking 2,000–3,000 mg daily for two weeks.

Pantothenic Acid for Virus Prevention

In addition to treating viral infections, pantothenic acid is also effective in preventing them. In *The Natural Health Guide to Beating the Supergerms,* Jack Challem and Richard Huemer, M.D., wrote that pantothenic acid is essential for the health of the thymus gland and antibody production. Antibodies are the scout molecules of the immune system that identify disease-causing intruders (like viruses, bacteria, and fungi) and stick to them. They alert immune-system cells to attack the foreign invaders and destroy them, thus preventing and controlling disease.

It is our opinion that it is more important to use pantothenic acid in the prevention of viruses in the winter because we need more of this molecule in cold temperatures. When the temperature drops, the body makes more coenzyme A, which is needed for heat production in the cells to help warm the body. The more coenzyme A that's made, the more pantothenic acid is used up. As a result, levels of pantothenic acid drop, and we become more susceptible to viral infections.

Pantothenic Acid's Effects on Heart Disease

It also has been suggested that pantothenic acid is helpful for heart disease. Michael Murry, N.D., and Joseph Pizzorno, N.D., in their book, *Encyclopedia of Natural Medicine,* recommended pantothenic acid in combination with carnitine and coenzyme Q_{10} for people with heart disease. This is because these supplements prevent the accumulation of fatty acids within the heart muscle. Pantothenic acid, along with alpha-lipoic acid and magnesium, has shown some promising results for cardiac patients.

Conclusion

Pantothenic acid is known as an "antistress" vitamin that, in turn, helps with the treatment and prevention of viruses. It is especially important to take pantothenic acid supplements in the winter, when our bodies use up more of this vitamin. In addition, pantothenic acid has been shown to be helpful in the prevention and treatment of heart disease.

CHAPTER 6

VITAMIN B$_6$
(PYRIDOXINE)

Vitamin B$_6$ (pyridoxine) is necessary for the metabolism of amino acids (the building blocks of proteins), carbohydrates, and fats, and the synthesis of neurotransmitters (the molecules that facilitate communication between nerve cells), red blood cells, enzymes, and hormones. Clinically, vitamin B$_6$ has many uses, which range from treating ringing in the ears, carpal tunnel syndrome, and migraine headaches to preventing heart disease and controlling asthma. Also, as you learned in the introduction to this book, it can be a life-saving treatment in the case of mushroom poisoning.

Sources of Pyridoxine

There are many natural sources of vitamin B$_6$. Chicken, beef, fish, and eggs are good animal sources, while spinach, carrots, avocados, bananas, certain nuts, alfalfa, and whole wheat are good plant sources.

How Much Pyridoxine Is Enough?

The RDA for vitamin B$_6$ is 2 mg. However, most people do quite well with 10–25 mg as part of a B-complex supplement. In most cases, people rarely need more than 100 mg of B$_6$ daily. If you feel you need more vitamin B$_6$, be sure to get the advice of a nutritionally oriented doctor who is very familiar with vitamin supplementation. In the case of vitamin B$_6$, more may not always be better. As opposed to most of the other water-soluble vitamins, too much vitamin B_6 can be toxic. In very high doses over the course of several months, pyridoxine may cause loss of muscle coordination and nerve damage. This vitamin should not be taken in single doses exceeding 100 mg. After taking a dose of 100 mg, another dose should not be taken for at least eight hours.

Maladies Due to Pyridoxine Deficiency

There are a wide variety of symptoms associated with vitamin B_6 deficiency. Initially, you would experience vague symptoms like insomnia, fatigue, and depressed mood, slow wound healing, and gastrointestinal distress. As this deficiency persists, blood disorders like anemia (low levels of red blood cells) and elevated blood lipids develop. Later, you would begin to develop inflammation of your tongue and mouth and then possibly display neurological symptoms such as paresthesias ("pins and needles") in the hands and feet, and, finally, seizures. The deficiency could also lead to kidney stones.

Pyridoxine's Effects on Migraines

Migraine headaches are a very common problem in our society. These headaches are likely caused by the temporary widening of the blood vessels in the brain and the resulting excessive pulsation of these vessels. Many migraine sufferers can pinpoint their migraine triggers, which may include stress, food allergies, food intolerances, flashing lights, and hormonal changes. Many studies have shown that by just removing offending foods from the diet, the incidence of migraines can be reduced by 40 to 70 percent. Common food triggers include chocolate, red wine, cheese, beer, cow's milk, wheat products, citrus fruit, and eggs. These foods either contain or increase the amount of histamine in the bloodstream, thus affecting the blood vessels in the brain. The enzyme that breaks down or degrades histamine requires pyridoxine to do its job. So, if you suffer from migraines, be sure to avoid offending foods, reduce the stress in your life, and consider supplementing your diet with reasonable doses of pyridoxine and riboflavin (see Chapter 3). A reputable and knowledgeable integrative or naturopathic doctor can help set up a personalized anti-migraine program for you if one is required.

Pyridoxine's Effects on Carpal Tunnel Syndrome

Carpal tunnel syndrome is another common problem that can be improved with vitamin B_6. This condition is especially prevalent among people who do work that involves repetitive motion of their hands—this makes secretaries, writers, assembly-line workers, and supermarket cashiers susceptible.

Many years ago, John Ellis, M.D., discovered that patients with carpal tunnel syndrome had low levels of vitamin B_6. He gave them 100 mg of vitamin B_6 daily for three months and found that the symptoms were improved in the majority of patients. Vitamin B_6 probably benefits this condition by stabilizing the nerves. By this same mechanism, vitamin B_6 has also been found to be useful in treating tinnitus, a condition of chronic ringing in the ears.

Pyridoxine's Effects on Insomnia

Insomnia is another common problem that many of us experience. In some cases, vitamin B_6 can help. This is because it stimulates the pineal gland in the brain to secrete increased amounts of melatonin, the sleep hormone. Interestingly, inadequate intake of vitamin B_6 can interfere with the ability to dream or recall dreams, which illustrates this vitamin's relationship to sleep. Conversely, too much vitamin B_6 can actually make a person's dreams so vivid that, in the morning, he or she feels tired.

Pyridoxine's Effects on Asthma

Vitamin B_6 is also beneficial in the treatment of some cases of asthma. Theoretically, this is because many people with asthmatic conditions have difficulty metabolizing the amino acid tryptophan and, therefore, have high levels of it. These high levels lead to higher levels of the brain chemical serotonin, which, along with its breakdown products, can worsen airway constriction. Supplementing with vitamin B_6 can improve tryptophan metabolism and, consequently, reduce the frequency and/or severity of asthma attacks.

Pyridoxine's Effects on Vascular Disease

The use of vitamin B_6 with other antioxidants has proven to be very helpful in vascular (blood vessel) disease. A study performed by Dr. Schnyder and associates used vitamin B_6, vitamin B_{12}, and folic acid to open closed blood vessels in patients after angioplasty procedures. One year after the initial procedure, they found that patients who were taking these vitamins along with their standard medications had lower risks of repeat angioplasties, nonfatal heart attacks, and death, when compared with those who were not taking the vitamins. This exciting study suggests that these vitamins may help prevent the progression of occlusive (clogged) artery disease. This may prove to be beneficial in a variety of serious diseases including heart disease, stroke, intermittent claudication (pain in the calves when walking because of clogged leg arteries), and even some cases of erectile dysfunction.

Vitamin B$_6$ is probably so effective in vascular disease because of its relationship to homocysteine. Homocysteine damages blood vessel walls and helps set the stage for cholesterol deposits. Homocysteine levels increase in a diet deficient in vitamin B$_6$ and folic acid. Today, there is more and more evidence that homocysteine is a cardiovascular risk factor as important as the better-known ones such as high cholesterol.

Homocysteine
A toxic breakdown product of methionine, an essential component of protein. It may have as much impact on your risk for heart disease as high cholesterol.

Vitamin B$_6$ and folic acid, as well as vitamin B$_{12}$ and choline, play vital roles in controlling homocysteine levels.

Pyridoxine's Effects on High Blood Pressure

Another cardiovascular disease in which vitamin B$_6$ has shown promise is hypertension, or high blood pressure. In one Turkish study, doctors gave twenty patients with high blood pressure vitamin B$_6$ daily for four weeks. At the conclusion of the study, most patients showed improvement in both their systolic (higher number) and diastolic (lower number) blood pressure.

Pyridoxine's Effects on Immune Suppression

Vitamin B$_6$ is essential to the proper function of the immune system. It helps stimulate the immune response and activates the synthesis of antibodies. People who have HIV or diabetes, or are on immune-suppressing medications like chemotherapy drugs, antirejection drugs, and some rheumatoid arthritis medications have depressed immune systems. To make matters worse, they often have low levels of vitamin B_6. People with very low vitamin B_6 levels also have low white blood cell counts. The body needs white blood cells to defend it against disease-causing organisms and cancer cells. Moreover, scientists have found that proper levels of pyridoxine are required for the proper function of the thymus, the site where many of the immune-system cells are programmed to do their jobs. For all these reasons, anyone whose body is immunosuppressed should be consuming sufficient amounts of vitamin B_6 daily.

Pyridoxine's Effects on Women's Health

Like folic acid, sufficient amounts of vitamin B_6 are most likely required during the prenatal period. In animals, pregnant females that were very low in vitamin B_6 were more likely to give birth to newborns that developed seizures and movement disorders. In humans, the newborn infants were more likely to develop neurological symptoms. Moreover, a vitamin-B_6 deficiency during pregnancy has been associated with cleft palates in newborns. Therefore, it's vitally important that women of childbearing age ensure that they are getting an adequate amount of the B vitamins by taking a B-complex capsule daily. There is also some evidence to suggest that pyridoxine can help relieve morning sickness.

Another women's health issue where pyridoxine is likely beneficial is in the treatment of cervical dysplasia and cervical cancer. As mentioned, pyridoxine is an essential substance for immunity against cancer, and it's important for the balance and metabolism of the female sex hormones. Studies on the preventative and healing potential of pyridoxine on estrogen-related cancers may shed some interesting light on this subject. Laboratory studies have already shown that vitamin B_6 stops the growth of liver cancer in tissue cultures.

Pyridoxine's Effects on Colon Cancer

Several studies have reported that the less vitamin B_6 you consume, the higher your risk is for colon cancer. One Japanese study examined the effect of dietary vitamin B_6 on the production of colon tumors in mice. One group of mice was fed a carcinogen (a cancer-causing agent) and given vitamin B_6, and a second group of mice was fed just the carcinogen. The vitamin B_6 group developed significantly fewer tumors than the mice that received just the carcinogen. The authors concluded that dietary vitamin B_6 suppressed colon-tumor formation by reducing the rate of cell division, reducing free radicals and thus reducing oxidative stress, and by discouraging the formation of new blood vessels leading to a tumor (angiogenesis).

Pyridoxine's Effects on Mushroom Poisoning

Mushrooms are the sexual fruiting body of a fungus. Fungi are unlimited chemical factories that can produce practically any drug or toxin. For example, fungi are responsible for synthesizing cyclosporine (an antirejection drug for transplant patients), aflatoxin (a most potent carcinogen), the active ingredient in Lipitor (a cholesterol-reducing drug), hepatotoxins (deadly poisons that destroy the liver), and many more.

An interesting therapeutic use of vitamin B_6 is as an antidote to *Gyromitra* mushroom poisoning. The North American version of this mushroom resembles a brain. It produces a water-soluble toxin that is identical in chemical structure to certain rocket fuels and can cause a rapid illness that can result in death. Lower doses of

Gyromitra toxins can cause a slow illness that can result in cancer. This toxin interferes with the metabolic production of vitamin B_6 and causes seizures, vomiting, cramps, diarrhea, liver destruction, and tumor formation.

Although fairly common among amateur mushroom hunters, most cases of poisoning with this mushroom are misdiagnosed, and about 15 percent of people that eat this mushroom die. Its toxin is so potent that even a chef cooking this mushroom can get sick just from inhaling the fumes. If this poisoning is diagnosed properly, intravenous vitamin B_6 is lifesaving.

Conclusion

As you can see, pyridoxine is essential to the normal function of the body. In addition to its vital role in maintaining basic processes in the body, vitamin B_6 has many clinical uses. These range from treating insomnia and migraine headaches to preventing heart disease and colon cancer. It is also an important prenatal supplement.

CHAPTER 7

FOLIC ACID
(FOLATE)

You've probably heard that the B vitamin folic acid (folate) is an important prenatal vitamin supplement. This is because it has been shown to prevent spinal cord, or neural tube, defects in infant development. In addition, folic acid plays an important role in other bodily processes, including the production of genetic material, energy, and red blood cells. It also helps metabolize proteins and, when used along with other B vitamins, decreases homocysteine levels to decrease the risk of heart disease.

Sources of Folic Acid

The name folic acid shares the Latin root "folium" with the word "foliage" because the vitamin was first extracted from spinach and other leafy green vegetables. In addition to being found abundantly in vegetables such as lettuce, spinach, beet greens, asparagus, and bean sprouts, it is also found in organ meats, including liver and kidney. Other good sources of folic acid include oranges, pineapples, cantaloupes, bananas, lima beans, green peas, whole wheat, and soybeans. This vitamin is very sensitive to heat, light, cooking, and even long-term storage at room temperature.

Recently, scientists have been trying to genetically engineer food crops to increase their folate levels. Plants can synthesize folate from another B-complex vitamin, para-amino benzoic acid (PABA), discussed in Chapter 10. Some researchers have actually removed folate-producing genes from bowel bacteria and implanted this genetic material into plant crops to increase their levels of folate.

Folic Acid Deficiency

Consequences of folic-acid deficiency include macrocytic anemia, low white blood cell counts, and sores in the gastrointestinal tract. Pregnant women who are deficient in folic acid are more likely to give birth to infants with neural tube defects, such as spina bifida.

Another theoretical, but potentially serious, effect of a severe deficiency in folic acid is the possible development of cancer. This is because folic acid is necessary for the production and repair of DNA. Consequently, a deficiency in folic acid may lead to irreparable DNA mutations, and this condition may lead to cancer. While there is a large amount of epidemiological evidence that supports the hypothesis that insufficient folic acid can promote the development of tumors, the data from case-control studies are less consistent, suggesting that further study is required.

Since folic acid is necessary for the production of white blood cells and antibodies, a deficiency of this vitamin can lead to a compromised immune system. When the immune system is not functioning properly, the body becomes vulnerable to infections, cancer, and other types of damaging stress.

How Much Folic Acid Is Enough

Folic acid is exceptionally safe. The adult RDA value for folic acid is 400 mcg (600 mcg in pregnant women). However, a daily dose of 400–800 mcg can lower homocysteine levels and presumably reduce the risk of cardiovascular diseases. A dose of 1 mg in a pregnant woman, especially in the first few weeks of pregnancy, will reduce the risk of neural tube defects. This is why it is very important that all women of childbearing age get sufficient amounts of folic acid.

While very safe overall, the only major concern about folic acid is that it may mask the symptoms of a vitamin B_{12} deficiency. This masking does not usually become an issue unless a person takes more than 5,000 mcg of folic acid daily for an extended period of time. It is easily avoided by also taking a small amount of vitamin B_{12}. Because these two vitamins work together, as do all of the B vitamins, it's once again probably the wisest decision to take the entire B complex as a single supplement.

Folic Acid's Effects on Cervical Dysplasia

Folic acid is an incredibly important vitamin for women. In addition to the well-documented daily need of 1 mg in pregnant women to prevent neural tube defects, folic acid could prove effective as part of the treatment plan for cervical dysplasia, a precancerous condition. Cervical dysplasia is caused by one of the human papilloma viruses, a sexually transmitted disease that is one of the most common viruses in people. It is also the virus that causes warts. There are usually no symptoms of cervical dysplasia, so regular Pap smears are essential for early detection.

Cervical Dysplasia

The abnormal growth of the epithelial tissue on the surface of the cervix.

Tori Hudson, N.D., of Portland, Oregon, has seen excellent results in treating cervical dysplasia with folic acid in tandem with a combination of other vitamins. She inserts vitamin suppositories into the cervix in order to put these healing nutrients in direct contact with the viral infection.

The word "plasia" suggests growth. Cervical

dysplasia is defined as disordered growth of the cells of the cervix. There are various stages of cervical dysplasia, which are determined by the amount of abnormal cells. These stages of dysplasia are mild (CIN I), moderate (CIN II), and severe (CIN III). Left untreated, this condition may develop into a dangerous invasive cancer.

If the dysplasia is high grade, it should be promptly treated with one of the surgical techniques suggested by your doctor. However, if your doctor tells you that it is low grade, it is not an emergency and you may have other choices. Many forms of low-grade viral dysplasia will spontaneously heal over a few months. With healthy life choices, it can be simply monitored with frequent Pap smears or with lab tests that determine the specific HPV virus causing the infection. With low-grade cervical dysplasia, folic acid supplementation, pyridoxine, beta-carotene, vitamin A, and certain other natural treatments have been found to have a high cure rate. See your integrative or naturopathic doctor prior to starting a nutritional program for cervical dysplasia. Interestingly, in the very near future, an anti-HPV vaccine should become available that has the potential to nearly eliminate the problem of cervical dysplasia for generations of women to come.

Folic Acid's Effects on Anemia

Anemia
A condition in which the body has a lower than normal red blood cell count, leading to paleness, weakness, and shortness of breath.

The body requires folic acid for the production of red blood cells. So it stands to reason that one of the more universally accepted roles of folic acid is in the workup and treatment of certain types of anemia. A measurement of folic acid is an important blood test for people with macrocytic anemia (low red blood cell count with larger than normal red blood cells). If folic acid levels are found to be low, folic acid in high doses daily is usually a standard treatment.

Folic Acid's Effects on Cancer

Studies have suggested that a diet rich in vegetables and fruit can protect a person against cancer, and as you know, eating proper amounts of these plant foods provide high levels of folic acid. However, a group of German scientists suggests that since there are only a few human intervention trials showing that folic acid specifically can modify and inhibit the development of cancerous tumors, additional studies are required in order to determine whether this vitamin is a useful agent in the prevention of cancer.

Nonetheless, a group of medical scientists from a large Eastern university studied folate levels in women and their corresponding chances of developing colon cancer. The group studied almost 90,000 nurses over several years who were cancer free in 1980 and followed them through 1994. More than 400 nurses developed colon cancer over that period. The researchers reported that the longer a nurse took folate, the lower her risk of developing colon cancer. Also, the group of women who took more than 400 mcg of folate each day had a 31 percent lower risk of developing cancer than a group who took only 200 mcg a day. Amazingly, the researchers found that women who took folate for fourteen years decreased their risk of developing colon cancer by 75 percent.

The researchers reported that, among other things, folate from both food and supplements can help a woman stay healthy but a higher dose of folate from capsule supplements appeared to work better.

Folic Acid's Effects on Familial Hyperlipidemia and Cystic Fibrosis

Some people take extra folic acid and vitamin B_{12} to theoretically minimize their DNA damage, which can also exacerbate heredity conditions such as familial hyperlipidemia (elevated lipids or cholesterol in the bloodstream) and cystic fibrosis (a functional disorder of the exocrine glands).

Folic Acid's Effects on Heart Attacks and Strokes

As you now know, homocysteine is a corrosive amino acid that is found in the bloodstream and can damage blood vessel walls and set up a cascade of events leading to heart attacks and strokes. Folic acid, in combination with vitamin B_6, choline, and vitamin B_{12}, plays a very important role in controlling homocysteine levels.

Stroke
A blockage of blood flow to areas of the brain that can cause paralysis, difficulty speaking, or other nerve problems. If the blockage lasts for a period of time, it can destroy brain tissue, which can make these changes permanent or even cause death.

You can protect yourself from homocysteine-induced strokes and heart attacks just by eating a good diet and taking a B-complex supplement. In our medical practice, we regularly see high homocysteine levels in patients who are having chest pain. Although they have seen a cardiologist and are taking several prescription drugs, the chest pain continues. We've found that their chest pain is often alleviated when they simply change their diets and take adequate B-vitamin supplements.

Conclusion

Folic acid is an abundant B vitamin in our food supply. Despite its wide availability, it may be necessary to supplement with it to ensure you're getting enough. Adequate intake is especially important in pregnant women to prevent serious birth defects. And since the body requires folic acid in its formation of red blood cells, supplementation with high doses is sometimes necessary in people with certain types of anemia. Folic acid has also been shown to reduce the incidence of colon cancer, heart attacks, and strokes. Along with the other B vitamins, this vitamin promotes good health and overall well-being.

CHAPTER 8

VITAMIN B_{12}
(COBALAMIN)

Probably the most complex of the B vitamin molecules, vitamin B_{12} is very large and is assembled around an atom of the metal cobalt. There are four known forms of vitamin B_{12} in humans—cyanocobalamin, methylcobalamin, hydroxycobalamin, and adenosylcobalamin.

Vitamin B_{12} is essential for life because it is required in the manufacturing of the nucleic acids that make up genes and for the production of energy from sugars and fats. It is also fundamental in the formation of red and white blood cells. Moreover, it's necessary for the normal growth of the nervous system and is vital in the formation of the myelin sheath (insulation material) around the nerves. In addition, the body requires this vitamin to manufacture the neurotransmitter acetylcholine, and thereby helps nerves communicate with one another and with the brain.

Nucleic Acids
The building blocks of genetic material. Found in the fungal, animal, bacterial, and plant kingdoms.

The absorption of vitamin B_{12} by the small intestine is dependent on a chemical that is secreted by the stomach called "intrinsic factor" (IF). IF combines with vitamin B_{12}, and the resulting complex can then pass through the wall of the small intestine and into the bloodstream. Vitamin B_{12}

Intrinsic Factor (IF)
A substance produced by the lining of the stomach and intestines that is essential for the absorption of vitamin B_{12}.

also works hand in hand with vitamin C in the process of absorption and digestion.

Sources of Vitamin B_{12}

Foods of animal origin, such as milk, cheese, fish, eggs, and meat are considered the only important food sources of vitamin B_{12}. Organ meats such as liver are especially packed with vitamin B_{12}. Thus, vegans (people who eat no animal products whatsoever) require dietary supplements of this vitamin. Vitamin B_{12} can be synthesized by microbes in the laboratory, which strict vegetarians and vegans may find acceptable as a source.

Vitamin B_{12} Deficiency

Vitamin B_{12} is considered a micronutrient (required in only very small amounts) because it is stored for up to nine months in the liver and kidneys. However, a surprisingly large portion of the population, even in highly developed nations, has been found to be deficient in vitamin B_{12}.

Up to 10 percent or more of senior citizens are estimated to be vitamin B_{12} deficient. In accordance with this fact, scientists have found that vitamin B_{12} levels decline with age. This may be due to reduced intake or unhealthy diets. Production of IF also declines with age, leading to decreased absorption of this vitamin.

To make matters worse, as many as one-third of people over age sixty-five suffer from a condition known as "atrophic gastritis." This inflammatory condition leads to the breakdown of IF and the malfunction of the acid-secreting stomach cells, making it even harder for the body to absorb vitamin B_{12}. These factors can cause a serious state of deficiency. To overcome this, a person may require injections of vitamin B_{12}, sublingual

Atrophic Gastritis
Long-term inflammation of the stomach.

(under the tongue) supplements, or both.

Vitamin B_{12} deficiency can lead to general symptoms such as fatigue, pale complexion, forgetfulness, and paresthesias ("pins and needles") of the hands and feet. However, the classic disease induced by a vitamin B_{12} deficiency is pernicious anemia. This disease is defined by a decreased amount of IF causing the inability to absorb vitamin B_{12} and, thus, a megaloblastic anemia (large individual red cells with a low total number of cells). If people don't produce enough hydrochloric acid (stomach acid), they also have difficulty absorbing vitamin B_{12}. The result of this condition is that a person will develop the fatigue and pale skin of anemia, but will also have a higher risk for esophageal cancer, which is extremely difficult to treat successfully.

Because vitamin B_{12} is required for normal cell division, it is especially necessary for the production of the rapidly and constantly dividing sperm cells. Men with low levels of vitamin B_{12} often have low sperm counts, poor sperm motility, and problems associated with infertility. (Incidentally, men with low sperm counts tend to be deficient in other antioxidant vitamins such as vitamins E and C, and the mineral selenium.)

How Much Vitamin B_{12} Is Enough?

The RDA of vitamin B_{12} is 2 mcg daily, which is too low to meet the needs of most people. In cases of poor absorption and poor production of intrinsic factor (IF), which controls vitamin B_{12} absorption, more vitamin B_{12} is required. The simplest way to counter absorption problems is to take a sublingual B_{12} tablet (placed under the tongue). The network of blood vessels under the tongue will readily and directly absorb the tablet. Taking B_{12} this way—or by injection administered by a doctor—bypasses the digestive system and the need for intrinsic factor. A dose of 100–500 mcg of vitamin B_{12} daily in the sublingual form is reasonable for most people. Excess doses are harmless and excreted.

Vitamin B_{12}'s Effects on Heart Health

Vitamin B_{12} is important for a healthy heart because of its relationship with homocysteine. When homocysteine becomes elevated in the bloodstream, it becomes a risk factor for cardiovascular disease. Supplementing with vitamin B_{12} can lower homocysteine levels and lower the risk for heart attacks and strokes. In one study, a Canadian group of researchers followed thirty-eight men and women for more than four years. The group was supplemented with vitamin B_{12}, folic acid, and vitamin B_6. This supplemental regimen lowered homocysteine levels and reduced the subjects' risk of heart disease.

Vitamin B_{12}'s Effects on Immune Function

Vitamin B_{12} is necessary for normal immune function. Without enough vitamin B_{12}, the body's production of white blood cells can decrease, and white blood cell behavior may become abnormal. White blood cells are the "scout soldiers" of the immune system. They travel through the bloodstream and tissues in search of cancer cells and dangerous pathogens. These white blood cells are looking to identify and destroy these disease-causing entities. If there aren't adequate amounts of vitamin B_{12}, not only will fewer of these "scout soldiers" be produced, but the white blood cells that exist cannot function to their full ability and the immune system becomes compromised.

Pathogens
Organisms such as bacteria, viruses, and parasites that cause disease.

The fact that a vitamin B_{12} deficiency causes a

state of immunodeficiency is especially dangerous for people with AIDS whose immune systems are already compromised. To worsen the
situation, people with AIDS have a tendency to
have lower vitamin B$_{12}$ levels than normal. This
may occur as a result of decreased absorption of
the vitamin, reduced ingestion, or depletion of
the vitamin by antiviral medications.

It is also true that as AIDS progresses, blood
levels of vitamin B$_{12}$ fall further. Additionally, vitamin B$_{12}$ inhibits reproduction of the HIV virus in
cell-culture studies, and in the future it may be
one of the standard components of a good therapeutic regimen for AIDS.

Another specific group of people who likely
need vitamin B$_{12}$ supplementation are those
who have Crohn's disease. Crohn's disease is a
painful inflammatory bowel disease that can
cause damage to any part of the digestive tract.
Many cases involve the mid-part of the small
intestines. This disease can destroy the wall of
the intestines, sometimes even forming deep
ulcers that can evolve into penetrating holes,
called "fistulas." A healthy mid-intestine is vital
for B$_{12}$ absorption. Thus, people with Crohn's
are often vitamin B$_{12}$ deficient and require supplementation.

Vitamin B$_{12}$'s Effects on Multiple Sclerosis

Vitamin B$_{12}$ is important in the formation and
maintenance of the myelin sheath that surrounds
nerves and allows electrical impulses to travel
quickly along nerves. Without sufficient myelination of the nerves, electrical signals from the
brain cannot reach the proper destination and
the consequences of this can range from partial
or total paralysis to loss of touch sensation or
loss of eyesight.

This concept of insufficient myelination of

nerves is the cause of multiple sclerosis (MS). While we still don't know the exact cause of MS, some microbiologists believe that the initial damage to the nerve sheath is caused by a herpes virus and further damage is produced by the person's own overactive immune system.

Since vitamin B_{12} is critical to the maintenance of the myelin sheath, deficiencies in this vitamin can cause symptoms similar to MS. Some scientists have even reported that high doses of vitamin B_{12} may increase brain function and improve eyesight in MS patients, but don't appear to reverse the paralysis. Vitamin B_{12} blood levels should be checked in anyone who is experiencing the symptoms of MS. If MS is found, a regular course of vitamin B_{12} shots by a doctor may help.

Vitamin B_{12}'s Effects on Memory

As seen in MS patients, some patients have reported that they can think more effectively and have improved memory when they receive vitamin B_{12} supplementation. It may not work the same way for everyone, but if you forget a lot of things, it's worth a try. One study found that older people with dementia were deficient in vitamin B_{12} and some of them exhibited sharper mental functioning with supplementation.

Vitamin B_{12}'s Effects on Allergies and Asthma

People often develop allergic symptoms and asthma from eating food that is treated with sulfites as preservatives. An Italian group of scientists found that supplementing with vitamin B_{12} blocked the sulfite-induced asthma in four of five children who ate this food.

Vitamin B$_{12}$'s Effects on Dandruff and Skin Conditions

Another very common condition in which vitamin B$_{12}$ may be helpful is dandruff. There is a great amount of anecdotal information suggesting that vitamin B$_{12}$ is helpful in the treatment of not only dandruff, but also many other skin conditions including forms of eczema. Some patients have reported great success with vitamin B$_{12}$. This may be due to its involvement, along with choline, in the production of a beneficial skin substance called "tetrahydrofolate." This possibility should be further studied, but the treatment would have a miniscule risk of negative side effects and may prove to be beneficial.

Conclusion

Vitamin B$_{12}$ is essential for life. Your body needs it to make genes and produce energy and blood cells. Because it is necessary to the formation of the myelin sheath (insulation material) around your nerves, deficiencies in this vitamin can cause symptoms similar to multiple sclerosis. High doses of vitamin B$_{12}$ may increase brain function and improve eyesight in people with MS. In addition, it is important to take sufficient amounts of B$_{12}$ for a healthy heart and vital immune system.

CHAPTER 9

CHOLINE AND INOSITOL

Choline was not classified officially as an essential B vitamin until 1998. It forms the core of a key neurotransmitter, acetylcholine, which is needed for thinking, moving, feeling, and most other functions coordinated by the nervous system. Inositol is another B vitamin that is involved in the health of cell membranes, liver function, and normal immunity. Let's take a look at choline first, and then we'll turn our attention to inositol.

Sources of Choline

Eggs and soybeans are rich sources of choline. However, cooking can destroy a large part of their vitamin content. To some extent, choline can be made by the "good" bacteria that reside in the intestines. Although choline is found in every cell, it is found in especially high amounts in lecithin, a type of phospholipid. Phospholipids, of which there are numerous types, are fat-soluble molecules with water-soluble tails that form the membranes of cells.

Lecithin
A yellow phospholipid that is essential for the metabolism of fats.

Lecithin is important in the health of the heart, blood vessels, nerve cells, and liver. Moreover, it has an important role in emulsification—a process by which fats become soluble in water. This process is necessary for the absorption of fat. Choline-rich lecithin enables bile (a liquid made by the liver and released by the gallbladder into the intestines) to absorb thiamine, cholesterol, fats, and fat-soluble vitamins. Without proper amounts of choline, the body would be unable to absorb these fat-soluble molecules, which could lead to a deficiency in the fat-soluble vitamins.

The food industry often adds lecithin to products such as margarine, mayonnaise, chocolate, and baked goods to reduce stickiness.

Choline Deficiency

Because choline is found in every living cell and the body produces some choline, severe deficiencies in this vitamin are rare. However, a severe choline deficiency would result in death since all cell membranes would literally fall apart without it.

Choline and Brain Function

Studies have shown that inadequate levels of choline in developing brains result in increased cell death. Therefore, adequate choline is needed for normal brain development. Because of this fact, it is important that pregnant women, and maybe even infants, get adequate amounts of choline. One study found that giving choline to young animals improved their memory and mental performance.

Since choline is so important to the nervous system, it makes sense that it may be useful in treating people with neurological disease. Some doctors have speculated that it may be helpful in treating Alzheimer's disease, but the results of studies have not provided a clear answer. While it seems to help in some patients, it does not help in others. The reason is probably related to the complicated nature of Alzheimer's disease.

Some neurologists think that the leakage of choline from brain cells may be a factor in the development of Alzheimer's disease. An abnormal molecule called "beta-amyloid protein" is found in the brains of Alzheimer's patients. As increased amounts of beta-amyloid appear, more choline is probably squeezed out of affected cells. This causes a reduction in the amount of acetylcholine and, consequently, a decline in brain function.

It's not a good idea to depend solely on choline to reduce the risk of Alzheimer's disease. Choline should, at the very least, be combined with vitamin B_{12} and carnitine. Even so, the most important factors in preventing or prolonging the onset of Alzheimer's disease are keeping a healthy lifestyle and an intellectually active brain.

Carnitine
An amino acid that is necessary for the processing of fats and for the production of energy from food.

Another way choline is important to the brain is when brain cells are exposed to periods of low oxygen, as in a stroke. Strokes are caused when blood flow to brain cells is cut off. This happens when blood vessels of the brain bleed or when a clot forms in a brain artery. A stroke is to the brain what a heart attack is to the heart, giving it the alternate name "brain attack." When a stroke, or brain attack, happens, brain cell membranes can break and choline leaks out of cells.

The well-known herb *Ginkgo biloba* has been reported to curb the breaking of cell membranes and help keep choline in brain cells. This may help minimize the devastating brain damage that often results from strokes, if given quickly. This will have to be studied more to see if these reports pan out.

You can see why proper amounts of choline are so important to brain function. Certain medications counteract choline to some extent and therefore are called "anticholinergic drugs." These medications can be very important in treating people with certain medical conditions, but they should be used with great care in patients with Alzheimer's disease. Medications that have anticholinergic properties include antihistamines such as Benadryl and Claritin. While these medications are lifesavers for people with terrible allergies, they can make people with Alzheimer's disease even more confused and should only be used under a doctor's supervision in any case of neurological diseases.

Choline Beyond the Brain

Choline is also involved in liver health in two major ways. First, as an emulsifier, choline is thought to be helpful in dissolving some of the fat stored in the liver. It's been shown that when a person with a damaged fatty liver is given oral choline, the fat content falls.

Second, it has been demonstrated that a choline-deficient diet can induce the development of liver cancer in some animals. In fact, when liver cells are grown in culture and deprived of choline, the normal programmed death of cells is altered. Normal cells live to a certain age and through a certain number of replications and then commit "cell suicide," in a process known scientifically as "apoptosis." Cancer occurs when the normal mechanism of apoptosis is broken and cell division goes haywire. Some researchers think that a deficiency of choline may interfere with the normal life and death cycles of cells and can lead to the development of cancer.

Inositol

Inositol is another B vitamin that has many functions in the body. It can be found in sufficient amounts in whole grains, fruits, meats, dairy products, and yeast cells. Since it is plentiful in many different foods, a naturally occurring inositol deficiency has never been found in humans.

In mice, a lack of inositol results in visual defects, neurological disease, hair loss, and growth failure. It is always hard to say if animal studies will correlate to humans, but it is reasonable to think that an inositol deficiency in people would lead to similar conditions.

One factor that can lead to a decreased amount of inositol in the body is alcoholism. Many chemical messengers in the brain require inositol-containing substances to operate. Large quantities of alcohol interfere with the production of these substances and can eventually lead to difficulties with memory and behavior as well as other mental problems. Massive alcohol intake not only depletes inositol, but many other B vitamins. For this reason, every time an inebriated person comes to the emergency room, they are given an IV "banana bag," which contains a mixture of multivitamins, including folic acid, thiamine, and inositol.

Therapeutic Uses of Inositol

There are many potential medical uses of inositol. It can be used to lower cholesterol levels, help restore injured skin, prevent artery disease, and protect the heart. However, some of the most interesting recent developments relate to inositol's role in treating psychiatric disorders. Doctors have found that high doses of inositol appear to be very effective in reducing depression, panic attacks, and obsessive-compulsive behavior. The effective dose for these conditions seems to be above 1 gram per day.

Inositol in the form of inositol hexaphosphate (or IP-6) is showing some promising results in cancer research. Some studies using cell cultures and small animals have shown that in these models IP-6 is helpful in preventing or retarding the growth of cancer cells. Although this is promising, no human studies have been conducted.

Time will tell through further study if this information will show that IP-6 is helpful in treating cancers in people.

Inositol and Choline Together

Used together, inositol and choline seem to be clinically effective in treating premenstrual syndrome (PMS). Years ago, Carlton Fredricks, Ph.D., recommended that women with high estrogen profiles take these two supplements. He believed that they help the liver break "industrial strength" estrogen down into estriol, a more benign form of the hormone. The two vitamins seem to work for some women with PMS, perhaps by this mechanism. In treating PMS, women should take supplements of both inositol and choline in addition to a regular B-complex supplement.

As with all vitamins, dosages for choline and inositol should be tailored for a particular condition. If you have a condition that may require inositol or choline supplementation, you should eat foods rich in these vitamins or see a health professional who understands their effect on human physiology in order to suggest a proper supplement dose. However, supplements generally contain 250 mg each of choline and inositol, which appears to be a safe and adequate amount.

Conclusion

Though they do not receive much attention, choline and inositol can be very helpful for various conditions. Because choline is needed for normal brain development, it is important that pregnant women get adequate amounts of choline. Choline also may be helpful in treating Alzheimer's disease and in preventing cancer.

Inositol can be used therapeutically to lower cholesterol levels, restore injured skin, and protect the heart, and most recently, doctors have found that high doses of inositol appear to be very effective in reducing depression, panic attacks, and obsessive-compulsive behavior. Used together, inositol and choline seem to be clinically effective in treating premenstrual syndrome (PMS).

CHAPTER 10

BIOTIN AND PARA-AMINO BENZOIC ACID (PABA)

You may have seen biotin and para-amino benzoic acid (PABA) listed on shampoos, sunscreens, and beauty products. In addition to their glamorous promises to provide healthy skin, hair, and nails, they are important to overall health in many ways. Biotin is essential to metabolizing fats and may be useful in the treatment of type 2 diabetes. PABA is necessary for the body to metabolize amino acids and form blood cells. It may be helpful in treating osteoarthritis. Both are beneficial to good health as well as beauty.

Biotin

Biotin helps the body break down old fats and create new ones. Scientists at the University of Iowa found that people who don't get proper amounts of biotin have abnormal fatty acid and cholesterol metabolism. The effect of this B-complex vitamin on fatty acid and cholesterol metabolism explains the occurrence of loss of hair, skin rashes, and neurological disease that people with biotin deficiency develop. In addition, brittle nails often appear to be associated with a biotin deficiency. Doctors in New York administered 1,000 mcg of biotin to people who had brittle nails and most found this regimen to be helpful.

Biotin plays an important role in making proteins from amino acids and helps manufacture certain building blocks of genes. It is also necessary in the normal development of white blood cells that fight germs and destroy cancer cells. Because of this, low biotin levels can lead to a weakened immune system.

Sources of Biotin

Biotin is found in relatively small amounts in most natural foods. Higher amounts of biotin can be found in organ meats, egg yolks, natural whole grains, milk products, and fungal products like brewer's yeast. As with choline, the normal bacteria that live in the intestines usually produce satisfactory amounts of biotin. Because a healthy amount of biotin in the body has to do with healthy bacteria in the intestines, vegetarians are rarely deficient in biotin. (Vegetarians tend to eat a lot of fermented foods that are rich in beneficial bacteria, which produce lots of biotin.)

It is interesting to note that although egg yolks contain a particularly high amount of biotin, people who eat a lot of raw eggs can end up with a biotin deficiency. This is because raw egg whites contain a chemical called "avidin," which does not allow the body to absorb biotin. Cooking the eggs destroys avidin in the egg whites, allowing for the absorption of the biotin in the yolks.

Although it is unlikely that you eat very many raw eggs, everyone eventually gets older. It seems that some older people are deficient in biotin. Japanese scientists studied several hundred people over age sixty five and found that while some of the participants had normal biotin levels, others had very low levels. The scientists concluded that blood biotin levels in senior citizens vary greatly. Part of the problem is that as a person gets older, the gastrointestinal tract absorbs nutrients less efficiently. This makes eating a high-quality diet and taking supplements especially important for older people.

Biotin Deficiency

A deficiency in biotin can lead to many of the same symptoms of other B-vitamin deficiencies. Some of these symptoms include anemia, pale skin, poor appetite, and muscle pain. Additionally, people may experience flaking skin, paresthesias ("pins and needles") in their fingers and toes, and a sore tongue (glossitis).

If you take antibiotics several times a year, it may be wise to supplement with about 400 mcg of biotin daily. This is because antibiotics kill the good bacteria in your gut as well as the disease-causing bad bacteria. It is probably also a good idea to take acidophilus capsules or eat fresh yogurt while on antibiotics to replenish the normal intestinal bacteria.

Biotin's Therapeutic Effects

One area where biotin may be helpful therapeutically is in the treatment of type 2 diabetes mellitus (non-insulin dependent diabetes, formerly called "adult-onset" diabetes). Scientists have shown that biotin supplementation can increase cells' sensitivity to insulin. This helps the body use sugar more efficiently and lowers the levels of blood glucose, which causes many of the complications of diabetes.

Scientists in Japan studied biotin levels in patients with type 2 diabetes. They found that patients with high blood sugars often had low biotin levels. The scientists administered relatively high levels of biotin to these people and found that their blood sugar levels fell to almost one-half of their earlier levels. Biotin supplementation can be used in addition to a good diabetic regimen that is closely monitored by a doctor.

How Much Biotin Is Enough?

No cases of biotin poisoning have been described and no adverse effects of high dose administration of up to 10 mg for six months have been reported. So, an adult oral dose of up to 2,000 mcg (2 mg) each day appears to be safe and effective. The RDA for biotin is 300 mcg.

PABA

PABA doesn't stand for the Pan Asian Boxing Association as you might think; it stands for para-amino benzoic acid, another important B vitamin. The body requires PABA to metabolize amino acids, which come together to form proteins. PABA also functions in the formation of blood cells. It is found in foods like organ meats, wheat germ, whole grains, eggs, and brewer's yeast.

PABA as a Skin and Hair Aid

Known for its antioxidant properties, you may notice it as an ingredient in many sunscreens, because it can potentially block ultraviolet light from reaching the skin. PABA was actually the first true sunscreen that was widely available to the public and was popular in sunscreens from the 1950s through the 1970s. The problem with these early sunscreens is that many people have allergic reactions to PABA and its derivatives when applied topically to the skin. PABA is also notorious for staining clothes. There are now many known ingredients that are even more potent sun blockers than PABA and do not cause as much in the way of allergic reactions or clothes staining. Because of this, PABA is not as commonly used in sunscreens anymore.

Some information also exists that it may be useful in treating osteoarthritis and in helping with skin revitalization. In some people, it has also been shown to restore graying hair to its natural color. This is one reason that you will see it on the labels of many shampoo bottles and other hair products.

How Much PABA Is Enough?

There is no RDA for PABA. A dose of 50 mg per day is considered safe. At very high doses, however, PABA can cause some damage to the liver. Some people have also reported nausea and vomiting or allergic-type symptoms from taking PABA. In very large doses, PABA could also diminish the effectiveness of the very commonly used sulfa antibiotics.

Conclusion

There do not seem to be many circumstances in which a person will have to take very large doses of biotin or PABA. As a result, it is probably sufficient to take the amount that comes in a B-complex supplement. Of course, a doctor who knows your medical history personally may recommend higher doses for you. Still, biotin and PABA are essential B vitamins, and you should be sure to get them in adequate amounts in a B-complex supplement.

CHAPTER 11

ALPHA-LIPOIC ACID: A FORMER B VITAMIN

Alpha lipoic acid (ALA), also known as thioc-tic acid and sometimes simply as lipoic acid, is a vitamin-like substance that was once considered a B vitamin. The highest amounts of ALA are found in organ meats such as beef liver and kidney.

The body can use ALA as a cofactor (a helper molecule) in many important enzymatic process-es that involve the B vitamins. In addition, ALA is a very powerful antioxidant that is soluble in fat and somewhat in water, so it helps clear up excess free radicals, which can lead to aging and disease. ALA is sometimes called the "universal antioxidant" because it enhances the function of other antioxidants such as vitamins E and C.

In Dr. Burt Berkson's practice, many patients with diseases ranging from hepatitis C to dia-betic neuropathy are benefitting from the use of supplemental ALA.

The B Vitamin Connection

Both ALA and the B vitamins are essential in helping the cells' mitochondria make energy. When the mitochondria function correctly, they require a number of enzymes.

ALA is the major key that turns on these en-zymes. Thiamine, niacin, riboflavin, biotin, and other B-complex vitamins are also involved in this system of enzymatic processes and become depleted as the mitochondria produce energy. Therefore, if a person supplements with ALA, he or she must also take at least one B-complex capsule with it. In other words, since ALA revs up mitochondrial activity and uses up B vitamins in the process, there's a chance a person can become deficient in many key B vitamins without proper supplementation.

Conclusion

ALA has exciting therpeutic potential in treating many different medical conditions that are beyond the scope of this book. It is important to remember that taking ALA depletes your body of B vitamins. Therefore, it is essential to take a B-complex vitamin whenever consuming ALA supplements.

CONCLUSION

Overshadowed by the other antioxidants, nutrients, and prescription drugs that you hear about all the time, the B-complex vitamins are vitally important to health. They are needed for the normal operation of your immune system, nervous system, respiratory system, detoxification system, and every other system in your body. We believe, and research confirms, that many physical and mental problems can be alleviated with the B-complex vitamins in therapeutic or optimal doses.

Because our modern diet doesn't always supply us with adequate amounts of these vitamins in optimal combinations, it may be important to supplement with a B-complex capsule daily. In some cases of disease, higher doses of one or two B vitamins may be necessary as recommended by a doctor who is familiar with vitamin supplementation. Remember, however, that a deficiency in one B vitamin may mean there's a deficiency in another. And because all of the B vitamins work together, don't take one at the expense of the others. A nutritionally oriented doctor can help you determine what's right for you. When safe and natural agents are used to promote good health, such as with B-vitamin supplementation, you can be sure that good medicine is at work. "B" healthy!

SELECTED
REFERENCES

Aybak M. et al. "Effect of oral pyridoxine supplementation on arterial blood pressure in patients with essential hypertension" *Arzneimittelforschung.* 1995;45: 1271–1273.

Berkson B. "A conservative triple antioxidant approach to the treatment of hepatitis C." *Medizinische Klinik.* 1999;94(Supp. 3) 84–89.

Komatsu S, Yanaka N, Matsubara K, Kato N. "Antitumor effect of vitamin B_6 and its mechanisms." *Biochim Biophys Acta.* 2003 Apr 11;1647(1–2): 127–130.

Kulkarni S, Lee AG, et al. "you are what you eat." *Surv Ophthalmol.* 2005 Jul-Aug;50(4):389–393.

Nandi D, Patra RC, Swarup D. "Effect of cysteine, methionine, ascorbic acid and thiamine on arsenic-induced oxidative stress and biochemical alterations in rats." *Toxicology.* 2005 Jul 1;211(1–2): 26–35.

Okada H, Moriwaki K, Kanno Y. "Vitamin B_6 supplementation can improve peripheral polyneuropathy in patients with chronic renal failure on high-flux haemodialysis and human recombinant erythropoietin." *Nephrol Dial Transplant.* 2000 Sep;15(9): 1410–1413.

Perumal SS, Shanthi P, Sachdanandam, P. "Augmented efficacy of tamoxifen in rat breast tumorigenesis when given along with riboflavin, niacin, and CoQ_{10}: effects on lipid peroxidation and antioxidants in mitochondria." *Chem Biol Interact.* 2005 Feb 28; 152(1):49–58.

Rall LC, Meydani SN. "Vitamin B_6 and immune competence." *Nutr Rev.* 1993 Aug;51(8):217–225.

Scalabrino G. "Cobalamin (vitamin B_{12}) in subacute combined degeneration and beyond: traditional interpretations and novel theories." *Exp Neurol.* 2005 Apr;192(2):463–479.

Schnyder G, Roffi M, Flammer Y, et al. "Effect of homocysteine-lowering therapy with folic acid, vitamin B_{12}, and vitamin B_6 on clinical outcome after percutaneous coronary intervention. The Swiss Heart Study: a randomized controlled trial." *JAMA* 2002;288(8):973–979.

Schoenen J, Lenaerts M, Bastings E. "Effectiveness of high-dose riboflavin in migraine prophylaxis: A randomized controlled trial." *Neurology* 1998;50: 446.

Seidman MD, Babu S. "Alternative medications and other treatments for tinnitus: facts from fiction." *Otolaryngologic Clinics of North America* 2003;2.

Strohle A, Wolters M, Hahn A. "Folic acid and colorectal cancer prevention: molecular mechanisms and epidemiological evidence." *Int J Oncol.* 2005 Jun;26(6):1449–1464.

OTHER BOOKS
AND RESOURCES

Berkson B., Challem J. and Heumer R. *Alpha-Lipoic Acid Breakthrough* (Random House/Prima, 1998).

Challem J. and Heumer, R. *The Natural Health Guide to Beating the Supergerms and Other Infections, Including Colds, Flu, Ear Infections and Even HIV* (Pocket Books, 1997).

Murray F. *100 Super Supplements for a Longer Life* (Keats Publishing, 2000).

Murray M. and Pizzorno J. *Encyclopedia of Natural Medicine* (Random House/Prima Publishing, 1998).

Rothfeld G. and Levert S. *Folic Acid and the Amazing B Vitamins: A Question-And-Answer Guide for Women and Men* (Berkley Publishing Group, 2000).

Ruben C. *Antioxidants: Your Complete Guide* (Random House/Prima 1995).

GreatLife Magazine
Consumer magazine with articles on vitamins, minerals, herbs, and foods.
Available for free at many health and natural food stores.

Let's Live Magazine
Consumer magazine with emphasis on the health benefits of vitamins, minerals, and herbs.
Customer service:
1-800-676-4333
P.O. Box 74908
Los Angeles, CA 90004
Subscriptions: 12 issues per year, $19.95 in the U.S.; $31.95 outside the U.S.

Physical Magazine

Magazine oriented to body builders and other serious athletes.

Customer service:

1-800-676-4333

P.O. Box 74908

Los Angeles, CA 90004

Subscriptions: 12 issues per year, $19.95 in the U.S.; $31.95 outside the U.S.

The Nutrition Reporter™ newsletter

Monthly newsletter that summarizes recent medical research on vitamins, minerals, and herbs.

Customer service:

P.O. Box 30246

Tucson, AZ 85751-0246

e-mail: jack@thenutritionreporter.com

www.nutritionreporter.com

Subscriptions: $26 per year (12 issues) in the U.S.; $32 U.S. or $48 CNC for Canada; $38 for other countries

INDEX

User's Guide to
Nutritional
Supplements

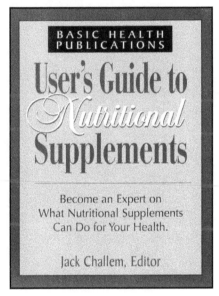

Everything You Need to Know to
Successfully Use the Most Popular
Vitamin, Mineral, and Herbal
Supplements to Improve Your Health

Jack Challem, Editor

336 pages • 8³/₈ x 10⁷/₈ • ISBN: 1-59120-067-9